HOW TO MAINTAIN A CONSISTENT DIABETES MANAGEMENT ROUTINE

ESSENTIAL ROLE OF CONSISTENCY IN PREVENTING COMPLICATIONS AND MAINTAINING OVERALL HEALTH AND DAILY BLOOD GLUCOSE , INSULIN AND MEDICATION

Meckwerey Zmpheria

TABLE OF CONTENT

INTRODUCTION

Diabetes is a persistent condition that influences hundreds of thousands of humans global. Managing diabetes effectively calls for a multifaceted method that encompasses weight-reduction plan, exercise, medication, and everyday monitoring of blood sugar stages. Whether you have Type 1, Type 2, or Gestational Diabetes, keeping a consistent management ordinary is crucial for preventing complications and accomplishing an awesome quality of existence.

In this book, "How to Maintain a Consistent Diabetes Management Routine," we purpose to offer you with realistic techniques, recommendations, and insights that will help you construct and maintain an powerful each day ordinary for handling your diabetes. By following the steering provided, you may benefit higher manipulate over your blood sugar levels and enhance your overall health and health.

GOALS OF THE BOOK

The number one purpose of this e-book is to equip you with the understanding and gear needed to create and preserve a regular diabetes control ordinary. By breaking down the various aspects of diabetes care into possible additives, we are able to assist you understand the significance of each element and how they work together to help your health.

1. Educate at the Fundamentals of Diabetes Management: We will provide a complete evaluate of what diabetes is, the distinctive forms of diabetes, and the significance of blood sugar manage.

2. Establishing a Daily Routine: Learn how to structure your day with constant exercises for monitoring blood sugar, taking medicinal

drugs, making plans meals, and incorporating physical activity.

3. Balanced Diet and Nutrition: Gain insights into creating balanced meals, knowledge the effect of various meals on blood sugar ranges, and handling weight loss plan successfully even when at the move.

4. Exercise and Physical Activity: Discover the blessings of regular exercising, sorts of physical sports suitable for diabetes, and the way to combine them into your each day routine.

5. Medication Management: Understand the various kinds of diabetes medicines, right utilization, handling aspect outcomes, and hints for visiting with medicine.

6. Monitoring Blood Sugar Levels: Learn the significance of regular blood sugar tracking, the way to use monitoring devices,

interpret readings, and maintain an accurate log e-book.

7. Stress Management and Mental Health: Explore the effect of stress on diabetes, techniques for stress reduction, and maintaining intellectual health.

8. Building a Support System: Recognize the position of family, pals, and healthcare vendors in helping diabetes control, and discover resources for extra guide.

9. Overcoming Common Challenges: Identify and address commonplace barriers along with diabetes burnout, dealing with ill days, and dealing with social conditions.

10. Adapting to Life Changes: Learn the way to control diabetes throughout primary existence activities and long term strategies for adapting to adjustments as you age.

EXPLANATION OF DIABETES AND ITS
KINDS (TYPE 1, TYPE 2,
GESTATIONAL)

EXPLANATION OF DIABETES AND ITS
TYPES

What is Diabetes?

Diabetes is a persistent clinical condition characterized through high ranges of glucose (sugar) in the blood. This takes place because the body either can not produce enough insulin or can't efficiently use the insulin it produces. Insulin is a hormone produced by means of the pancreas that facilitates glucose enter the cells to be used for electricity. Without enough insulin characteristic, glucose accumulates within the bloodstream, main to diverse health complications.

TYPES OF DIABETES

There are numerous forms of diabetes, with Type 1, Type 2, and Gestational Diabetes being the maximum commonplace. Each type has awesome causes, danger elements, and control approaches.

TYPE 1 DIABETES

Overview

Type 1 diabetes is an autoimmune circumstance in which the body's immune gadget mistakenly assaults and destroys the insulin producing beta cells in the pancreas. This outcomes in little to no insulin production, requiring individuals to depend upon insulin therapy for survival.

Causes

Genetic factors: A predisposition to Type 1 diabetes can run in households.

Environmental triggers: Certain viral infections or other environmental elements may additionally trigger the onset of Type 1 diabetes in genetically susceptible individuals.

SYMPTOMS

- Increased thirst and frequent urination
- Extreme starvation
- Unintended weight loss
- Fatigue and weak spot
- Blurred imaginative and prescient

MANAGEMENT

- Insulin remedy: Daily insulin injections or an insulin pump to control blood glucose tiers.
- Blood sugar monitoring: Regular monitoring of blood sugar ranges to modify insulin dosage and weight-reduction plan.
- Healthy consuming: A balanced food regimen to assist manipulate blood sugar ranges.
- Physical interest: Regular exercising to enhance insulin sensitivity and usual health.

TYPE 2 DIABETES

Overview

Type 2 diabetes is the maximum common shape of diabetes, accounting for about 9095% of all cases. It typically develops in adults over the age of forty five, but it's miles more and more visible in more youthful individuals, inclusive of kids and teenagers. In Type 2 diabetes, the body will become immune to insulin or the pancreas cannot produce enough insulin to hold regular blood glucose ranges.

Causes

- Genetic elements: A family records of Type 2 diabetes will increase the threat.
- Lifestyle elements: Obesity, physical inaction, and terrible food plan are good sized chance factors.
- Age: The threat increases with age, specially after age forty five.

- Other factors: Conditions such as high blood pressure and high cholesterol additionally growth the hazard.

SYMPTOMS

- Increased thirst and frequent urination
- Increased hunger
- Unintended weight reduction or weight gain
- Fatigue and weakness
- Blurred imaginative and prescient
- Slow healing sores and common infections

MANAGEMENT

- Medication: Oral medicinal drugs and on occasion insulin or other inject able medicines to assist manipulate blood glucose stages.
- Blood sugar monitoring: Regular tracking to tune blood sugar tiers and alter remedy as wanted.

- Healthy ingesting: A balanced food regimen low in subtle sugars and saturated fat.

- Physical interest: Regular exercise to enhance insulin sensitivity and aid weight control.

- Weight management: Achieving and keeping a wholesome weight to lessen insulin resistance.

GESTATIONAL DIABETES

Overview

Gestational diabetes develops in the course of being pregnant and commonly is going away after the baby is born. It takes place while the frame can't produce enough insulin to fulfill the elevated wishes throughout pregnancy, leading to high blood sugar degrees. Women who expand gestational diabetes are at better chance of growing Type 2 diabetes later in existence.

Causes

- Hormonal changes: Pregnancy hormones can intervene with the frame's capability to use insulin efficaciously.

- Risk elements: Being obese, having a family records of diabetes, or having had gestational diabetes in a preceding pregnancy boom the hazard.

SYMPTOMS

Gestational diabetes frequently does not purpose noticeable signs and symptoms. It is commonly detected via routine screening all through pregnancy.

MANAGEMENT

Blood sugar tracking: Regular tracking to make certain blood sugar ranges remain within the target variety.

- Healthy ingesting: A balanced weight-reduction plan tailored to the nutritional wishes of pregnancy and to manipulate blood sugar degrees.

- Physical pastime: Regular workout to help control blood sugar tiers.
- Medication: In a few instances, insulin or different medicines can be needed to manipulate blood sugar ranges.

IMPORTANCE OF MAINTAINING A CONSISTENT MANAGEMENT ROUTINE

Maintaining a constant management recurring is crucial for people with diabetes. Consistency in tracking, medicinal drug, eating regimen, and workout can help prevent headaches, enhance excellent of existence, and ensure usual well being.

1. Stabilizing Blood Sugar Levels

Preventing Fluctuations: Consistent control helps in retaining stable blood glucose tiers, stopping the highs and lows which can cause extreme headaches.

Avoiding Hypoglycemia and Hyperglycemia: Regular monitoring and

control reduce the threat of hypoglycemia
(low blood sugar) and hyperglycemia
(excessive blood sugar), each of which can
be dangerous if now not managed.

2. Reducing the Risk of Complications

 Short term Complications: Proper
management prevents immediate headaches
which includes diabetic KETOACIDOSIS
(DKA) in Type 1 diabetes and
HYPEROSMOLAR HYPERGLYCEMIC
state (HHS) in Type 2 diabetes.

 Long term Complications: Consistent
manage facilitates in stopping or delaying
long term headaches consisting of
cardiovascular ailment, nephropathy,
nephropathy, and nephropathy.

3. Enhancing Quality of Life

- Improving Energy Levels: Stable blood
  sugar tiers make a contribution to higher
  ordinary strength and much less fatigue,

enhancing every day functioning and productiveness.

- Mental Health Benefits: Effective diabetes management can lessen anxiety and stress associated with the condition, leading to stepped forward intellectual health and emotional wellness.

4. Facilitating Effective Medication Use

- Optimizing Medication Efficacy: Consistent workouts make certain that medicines, which include insulin, are taken as prescribed, optimizing their effectiveness in dealing with blood sugar stages.

- Reducing Side Effects: Proper timing and dosage adherence help in minimizing the facet outcomes related to diabetes medicines.

5. Promoting Healthy Habits

- Regular Physical Activity: Incorporating consistent workout routines helps improve insulin sensitivity, manage weight, and beautify cardiovascular health.

- Balanced Diet: Adhering to a regular meal agenda with balanced nutrients helps stable blood sugar ranges and ordinary health.

6. Enabling Better Data for Decision Making

- Tracking Patterns: Regular monitoring and logging of blood sugar ranges, eating regimen, and exercising offer precious facts to identify patterns and make knowledgeable modifications to the management plan.
- Informed Medical Consultations: Consistent records enables healthcare vendors make more accurate exams and offer personalized hints for better diabetes manage.

7. Building a Support System

 Involving Family and Friends: A regular ordinary permits circle of relatives and friends to understand and help your diabetes control efforts.

- Healthcare Team Collaboration: Consistency allows in preserving ordinary appointments and verbal exchange with healthcare companies, making sure ongoing assist and guidance.

8. Adapting to Changes and Challenges

- Managing Life Transitions: A well established habitual makes it simpler to adapt to changes which include journey, new process roles, or way of life modifications.

- Handling Stress and Illness: Consistent control gives a strong basis to better handle stress and contamination, minimizing their effect on blood sugar levels.

9. Empowering SelfManagement

Increasing Confidence: A steady recurring empowers individuals with diabetes to take manipulate of their circumstance, growing confidence in handling every day challenges.

Developing Discipline: Routine adherence fosters subject and responsibility, that are vital for long term diabetes management.

10. Improving Long term Outcomes

Extending Lifespan: Effective and steady diabetes control is related to an extended, healthier lifestyles by means of reducing the threat of excessive headaches.

Enhancing Quality of Life: Consistent control over diabetes interprets to a higher pleasant of life, permitting individuals to pursue their goals and experience regular activities without the steady burden of diabetes related issues.

CHAPTER ONE: UNDERSTANDING YOUR DIABETES

TYPES OF DIABETES

DETAILED REVIEW OF TYPE 1, TYPE 2, AND GESTATIONAL DIABETES

Understanding the unique styles of diabetes is essential for powerful control and treatment. we offer an in depth overview of Type 1, Type 2, and Gestational Diabetes, highlighting their reasons, signs, and management methods.

TYPE 1 DIABETES

Overview

Type 1 diabetes is an autoimmune circumstance where the frame's immune system assaults and destroys the insulin producing beta cells within the pancreas. As a end result, the frame produces little to no insulin, making people depending on insulin therapy.

Causes

Genetic Predisposition: A family records of Type 1 diabetes can increase the hazard.

Environmental Factors: Certain viral infections or environmental triggers can initiate the autoimmune response in genetically prone people.

Autoimmune Response: The frame's immune machine mistakenly objectives and destroys its insulin producing cells.

SYMPTOMS

- Increased Thirst: Excessive thirst despite drinking fluids.
- Frequent Urination: Increased urination, often noticed extra at night time.
- Extreme Hunger: Increased appetite without weight advantage.

- Unintended Weight Loss: Loss of weight notwithstanding consuming greater.
- Fatigue and Weakness: Persistent tiredness and lack of energy.
- Blurred Vision: Changes in imaginative and prescient because of high blood sugar tiers.
- Ketones in Urine: Presence of ketones, a byproduct of fat breakdown, in urine.

MANAGEMENT

- Insulin Therapy: Lifelong insulin injections or insulin pump to manage blood glucose ranges.
- Blood Sugar Monitoring: Frequent tracking of blood sugar stages to alter insulin and weight loss program.
- Healthy Eating: A balanced food regimen with controlled carbohydrate consumption.

- Regular Exercise: Physical pastime to enhance insulin sensitivity and common fitness.
- Education and Support: Diabetes training and help corporations for ongoing control.

TYPE 2 DIABETES

Overview

Type 2 diabetes is the maximum common form of diabetes, generally developing in adults over the age of forty five, though it's far increasingly seen in more youthful people, consisting of children and teens. It takes place when the body will become proof against insulin or while the pancreas cannot produce sufficient insulin to hold regular blood glucose stages.

Causes

- Genetic Factors: A own family records of Type 2 diabetes increases the chance.

- Lifestyle Factors: Obesity, physical state of no activity, and negative eating regimen are foremost individuals.

- Age: The hazard of Type 2 diabetes will increase with age.

- Other Health Conditions: Conditions such as high blood stress and high cholesterol levels also increase the hazard.

SYMPTOMS

- Increased Thirst and Urination: Frequent need to drink and urinate.

- Increased Hunger: Excessive starvation and eating.

- Unintended Weight Loss or Gain: Changes in weight without attempting.

- Fatigue and Weakness: Persistent tiredness.

- Blurred Vision: Vision adjustments because of fluctuating blood sugar levels.

- Slow Healing Sores: Wounds that take longer to heal.
- Frequent Infections: Increased susceptibility to infections.

MANAGEMENT

- Medication: Oral medicinal drugs, insulin, or other inject able medications to manipulate blood glucose ranges.
- Blood Sugar Monitoring: Regular monitoring to track levels and regulate remedy.
- Healthy Diet: Balanced meals with interest to portion sizes and carbohydrate content.
- Physical Activity: Regular exercising to enhance insulin sensitivity and manage weight.
- Weight Management: Achieving and maintaining a wholesome weight to reduce insulin resistance.

Regular Checkups: Ongoing hospital therapy to display and manage complications.

GESTATIONAL DIABETES

Overview

Gestational diabetes develops at some point of being pregnant and commonly resolves after childbirth. It occurs while the body cannot produce sufficient insulin to meet the multiplied needs at some point of pregnancy, leading to expanded blood sugar stages. Women who expand gestational diabetes are at better risk of growing Type 2 diabetes later in life.

Causes

- Hormonal Changes: Pregnancy hormones can intrude with the frame's capability to use insulin efficaciously.

- Risk Factors: Being obese, having a own family records of diabetes, or having had gestational diabetes in a preceding being pregnant will increase the threat.

- Insulin Resistance: Increased insulin resistance throughout being pregnant can cause gestational diabetes.

SYMPTOMS

Gestational diabetes often does no longer cause important signs and symptoms and is commonly detected via recurring screening during being pregnant. Symptoms, if present, may also consist of:

- Increased thirst and frequent urination
- Fatigue
- Nausea
- Blurred vision

MANAGEMENT

Blood Sugar Monitoring: Regular monitoring to ensure blood sugar tiers remain within the target range.

- Healthy Eating: A balanced weight loss plan tailor-made to the dietary desires of pregnancy and blood sugar control.
- Physical Activity: Regular exercise to help control blood sugar degrees.
- Medication: In some cases, insulin or other medicines can be needed to manage blood sugar ranges.
- Regular Prenatal Care: Frequent checkups to monitor the health of each mom and toddler.

THE IMPORTANCE OF BLOOD SUGAR CONTROL

Effective blood sugar manage is important for people with diabetes, as it performs a substantial role in stopping complications, keeping usual fitness, and improving first-class of existence. Proper management of blood glucose ranges involves a mixture of tracking, medication, weight loss plan, and way of life modifications.

1. Preventing Short Term Complications

Hypoglycemia

- Definition: Hypoglycemia takes place whilst blood sugar degrees drop too low, generally beneath 70 mg/dL.

- Symptoms: Symptoms consist of shakiness, sweating, confusion, irritability, and in intense cases, loss of awareness or seizures.

- Prevention: Regular monitoring and well timed consumption of carbohydrates can save you hypoglycemia, mainly while taking insulin or other diabetes medications.

HYPERGLYCEMIA

- Definition: Hyperglycemia happens when blood sugar tiers are too high, usually above a hundred and eighty mg/dL after food.

- Symptoms: Symptoms include elevated thirst, frequent urination, fatigue, and blurred vision.

- Prevention: Proper remedy adherence, dietary control, and exercise can assist prevent hyperglycemia.

2. Reducing the Risk of Long Term Complications

Cardiovascular Disease

- Impact: High blood sugar ranges can damage blood vessels and nerves, increasing the danger of heart disease and stroke.

- Control: Maintaining blood sugar within target stages reduces this threat, in conjunction with dealing with blood stress and cholesterol levels.

NEPHROPATHY

- Impact: Prolonged excessive blood sugar can cause nerve damage, leading to peripheral nephropathy (tingling, ache, or numbness in extremities) or autonomic nephropathy (affecting internal organs).

- Control: Keeping blood sugar ranges strong can prevent or sluggish the development of nephropathy.

Nephropathy

- Impact: Diabetes is a leading motive of kidney disorder. High blood sugar damages the blood vessels inside the kidneys, impairing their filtering ability.
- Control: Blood sugar manipulate, at the side of blood stress management, can shield kidney feature.

Retinopathy

- Impact: High blood sugar can damage the blood vessels inside the retina, leading to diabetic retinopathy, that could purpose vision problems and blindness.

- Control: Regular eye tests and blood sugar manipulate are critical in preventing and managing nephropathy.

3. Enhancing Quality of Life

Energy Levels

- Benefit: Stable blood sugar degrees contribute to greater regular energy degrees, reducing fatigue and improving every day functioning.
- Control: Balanced meals, ordinary physical activity, and right remedy use assist preserve strength.

Mental Health

- Benefit: Effective blood sugar control reduces strain and tension associated with diabetes, improving mental fitness.
- Control: Support from healthcare companies, diabetes schooling, and intellectual fitness resources can resource in dealing with mental influences.

4. Facilitating Effective Medication Use

Optimizing Treatment

- Benefit: Keeping blood sugar levels inside target levels facilitates medicines work extra efficiently.
- Control: Adhering to prescribed medicine regimens and tracking blood sugar regularly guarantees optimal treatment effects.

MINIMIZING SIDE EFFECTS

- Benefit: Proper blood sugar manipulate can lessen the hazard of medicine facet effects.
- Control: Following a consistent management plan allows mitigate potential adverse consequences.

5. Promoting Healthy Habits

Diet

- Benefit: A food regimen tailor-made to blood sugar manage promotes common health.

- Control: Eating balanced food with appropriate portion sizes and nutrient distribution helps solid blood sugar tiers.

Exercise

- Benefit: Regular physical pastime improves insulin sensitivity and aids in blood sugar control.

- Control: Incorporating steady exercising workouts helps control diabetes and enhances standard well-being.

6. Providing Valuable Data for Decision Making

TRACKING PATTERNS

- Benefit: Regular blood sugar tracking presents information to discover traits and make knowledgeable modifications.

- Control: Logging blood sugar degrees, meals intake, and workout enables tailor control strategies.

INFORMED HEALTHCARE DECISIONS

- Benefit: Accurate facts enables healthcare carriers to make better treatment hints.

- Control: Consistent monitoring and communication with healthcare groups make certain customized care.

7. Empowering SelfManagement

Confidence

- Benefit: Effective blood sugar manipulate builds confidence in dealing with diabetes.

- Control: Education, aid, and steady workouts empower individuals to take rate of their fitness.

DISCIPLINE

- Benefit: Adhering to a management plan fosters subject and accountability.

- Control: Structured routines and proactive control cause better long term consequences.

**Diet, exercise, remedy, and tracking
 Key Components of Diabetes
Management: Diet, Exercise, Medication,
and Monitoring**

Effective diabetes management relies on a comprehensive method that includes a balanced diet, regular exercise, appropriate remedy, and constant monitoring of blood sugar ranges. Each of these additives plays a essential role in preserving blood glucose inside target levels and preventing headaches.

 Diet

1. Importance of a Balanced Diet

- Blood Sugar Control: A balanced weight loss plan enables stabilize blood sugar degrees through controlling the intake of carbohydrates, which have the most immediately impact on blood glucose.

- Nutrient Intake: Ensures which you get essential vitamins, minerals, and vitamins important for overall health and well being.
- Weight Management: Helps in retaining a healthful weight, that's in particular essential for those with Type 2 diabetes.

2. Key Dietary Guidelines

- Carbohydrate Counting: Understanding and managing carbohydrate intake is vital. Choose complex carbohydrates over easy sugars.
- Portion Control: Monitor portion sizes to avoid overeating, which can lead to blood sugar spikes.
- Balanced Meals: Include a combination of macro nutrients—carbohydrates, proteins, and fat—in each meal.
- Low Glycemic Index Foods: Opt for ingredients with a low glycemic index,

that have a slower impact on blood sugar tiers.

- Regular Meal Times: Eating at normal duration helps prevent intense blood sugar fluctuations.

3. Recommended Foods

Whole Grains: Brown rice, oats, quinoa, and complete wheat products.

- Fruits and Vegetables: Non starchy greens like leafy veggies, peppers, and broccoli. Limit fruit consumption to manage carbohydrate load.

- Lean Proteins: Chicken, turkey, fish, tofu, and legumes.

- Healthy Fats: Avocados, nuts, seeds, and olive oil.

4. Foods to Limit or Avoid

Sugary Drinks and Sweets: Soda, sweet, and cakes.

- Processed Foods: High in dangerous fats, sugars, and sodium.

- Refined Carbohydrates: White bread, pasta, and rice.
- High Fat and Fried Foods: These can make contributions to weight benefit and insulin resistance.

Exercise

1. Importance of Physical Activity

Improved Insulin Sensitivity: Exercise helps the body use insulin greater correctly.

- Blood Sugar Control: Regular bodily interest can assist lower blood sugar ranges and enhance HbA1c.
- Weight Management: Aids in weight loss and keeping a wholesome weight.
- Cardiovascular Health: Reduces the threat of coronary heart ailment, which is a not unusual problem of diabetes.

2. Types of Exercise

- Aerobic Exercise: Activities like on foot, strolling, cycling, and swimming assist enhance cardiovascular fitness and blood sugar manage.

- Strength Training: Increases muscle tissues, which can improve insulin sensitivity and glucose uptake.
- Flexibility and Balance: Yoga and stretching exercises assist improve flexibility and save you damage.

3. Exercise Guidelines

- Frequency: Aim for at least 150 minutes of moderate intensity cardio exercise in keeping with week, spread over as a minimum 3 days.
- Consistency: Regular interest is extra beneficial than sporadic excessive workout routines.
- Monitoring: Check blood sugar ranges before and after workout, especially if taking insulin or medicinal drugs which could cause hypoglycemia.

- Hydration and Nutrition: Stay hydrated and have a snack handy to prevent low blood sugar.

Medication

1. Types of Diabetes Medications

Insulin: Required for Type 1 diabetes and occasionally for Type 2 diabetes. Various paperwork include rapid acting, short acting, intermediate acting, and long acting insulin.

Oral Medications: Common for Type 2 diabetes, along with metformin, sulfonamides, and DPP4 inhibitors.

Inject able Medications: Non insulin inflatables like GLP1 receptor agonists.

2. Importance of Adherence

- Effectiveness: Taking medications as prescribed ensures they work efficaciously to manipulate blood sugar tiers.

- Prevention of Complications: Proper medication use facilitates prevent each

short term and long term complications
of diabetes.

- Avoiding Side Effects: Following
  prescribed dosages minimizes the threat
  of aspect effects.

3. Tips for Medication Management

 Consistent Timing: Take medicinal drugs
on the identical time every day.

- Monitoring: Regularly display blood
  sugar ranges to assess medication
  effectiveness.

- Communication with Healthcare
  Providers: Report any aspect outcomes
  or worries to alter remedy as wished.

Monitoring

1. Importance of Blood Sugar Monitoring

- Immediate Feedback: Provides real time
  information on blood sugar tiers, helping
  you are making knowledgeable
  selections approximately weight loss
  plan, exercising, and medicinal drug.

- Long term Control: Regular monitoring facilitates music styles and trends, contributing to better long term diabetes management.

2. Tools for Monitoring

- Blood Glucose Meters: Portable gadgets for checking blood sugar levels.

- Continuous Glucose Monitors (CGMs): Devices that provide real time glucose readings for the duration of the day.

- A1C Tests: Measures common blood glucose stages over the last 23 months.

3. Monitoring Guidelines

- Frequency: The frequency of testing relies upon on the form of diabetes, the remedy plan, and individual wishes. Those on insulin may want to test extra frequently.

- Target Ranges: Work together with your healthcare company to determine your target blood sugar degrees.

CHAPTER TWO: SETTING UP A DAILY ROUTINE

CREATING A STRUCTURED SCHEDULE

THE IMPORTANCE OF CONSISTENCY IN DAILY ACTIVITIES FOR DIABETES MANAGEMENT

Consistency in each day sports is essential for effective diabetes management. A stable recurring facilitates hold blood sugar tiers within target ranges, reduces the chance of complications, and improves usual exceptional of existence.

1. Stabilizing Blood Sugar Levels

Predictable Patterns

- Benefit: Consistent exercises in food, exercise, and medicine result in predictable blood sugar patterns.
- Outcome: Easier to control and save you blood sugar spikes and drops.

MEAL TIMING

- Benefit: Eating meals and snacks at normal intervals helps keep constant blood sugar stages.

- Outcome: Prevents large fluctuations which can occur with irregular consuming habits.

EXERCISE ROUTINE

Benefit: Regular bodily hobby enables the frame use insulin more efficiently and maintains blood sugar degrees strong.

Outcome: Reduces the chance of surprising highs and lows.

MEDICATION ADHERENCE

Benefit: Taking medicinal drugs on the equal time every day guarantees steady blood sugar control.

Outcome: Maximizes the effectiveness of the drugs and minimizes aspect effects.

2. Reducing the Risk of Complications

Preventing Short Term Issues

- Benefit: Consistency facilitates keep away from acute complications like hypoglycemia (low blood sugar) and hyperglycemia (high blood sugar).
- Outcome: Reduces emergency conditions and maintains common fitness.

LONG TERM HEALTH

- Benefit: Regular control exercises help save you long term complications consisting of cardiovascular ailment, nephropathy, nephropathy, and retinopathy.
- Outcome: Enhances toughness and great of lifestyles.

3. Enhancing Quality of Life

ENERGY AND WELL BEING

- Benefit: Stable blood sugar levels contribute to extra constant energy levels and ordinary well-being.

- Outcome: Reduces fatigue and improves day by day functioning.

MENTAL HEALTH

- Benefit: Routine management reduces anxiety and strain associated with diabetes.
- Outcome: Improves intellectual health and emotional balance.

4. Facilitating Effective Medication Use

Optimal Medication Efficacy

- Benefit: Consistent timing and dosage adherence make sure medicines paintings correctly.
- Outcome: Better blood sugar manage and decreased risk of side effects.

REDUCING ADVERSE EFFECTS

- Benefit: Proper use of medicine reduces the chance of unfavourable consequences.
- Outcome: Enhances general treatment consequences.

5. Promoting Healthy Habits

Diet and Nutrition

- Benefit: Consistent ingesting behavior sell balanced nutrients and blood sugar control.

- Outcome: Supports usual fitness and well-being.

REGULAR PHYSICAL ACTIVITY

- Benefit: Consistent exercise exercises enhance insulin sensitivity and cardiovascular fitness.

- Outcome: Aids in weight control and standard physical fitness.

6. Providing Valuable Data for Decision Making

Tracking and Trends

- Benefit: Consistent monitoring gives dependable data to perceive developments and styles.

- Outcome: Enables knowledgeable adjustments to control strategies.

INFORMED HEALTHCARE DECISIONS

- Benefit: Accurate and constant facts assist healthcare companies make higher treatment recommendations.
- Outcome: Personalized and effective diabetes care.

MORNING ROUTINE

morning routine for effective diabetes management

Establishing a constant morning recurring is essential for people with diabetes. It units the tone for the day, helps hold strong blood sugar levels, and helps average health and wellness.

1. Wake Up at a Consistent Time

BENEFITS

- Regulates Blood Sugar: A regular wake up time enables adjust blood sugar degrees by preserving a regular time table for food and medicine.

- Enhances Sleep Quality: Regular sleep styles improve universal sleep satisfactory, that is vital for coping with pressure and blood sugar ranges.

TIPS

- Set an Alarm: Use an alarm clock to wake up on the identical time every day, even on weekends.

- Gradual Adjustments: If you want to change your wake up time, do it step by step in 15minute increments to permit your body to adjust.

2. Check Blood Sugar Levels

Benefits

- Informed Decisions: Knowing your blood sugar level inside the morning helps you make knowledgeable selections about your eating regimen, exercising, and remedy for the day.

- Immediate Action: Allows you to take on the spot movement in case your blood sugar is simply too excessive or too low.

TIPS

- Keep Supplies Handy: Have your glucose meter, test strips, and lancet device within clean reach.

- Record Results: Log your blood sugar readings in a diary or app to track styles and percentage together with your healthcare issuer.

3. Take Medication

BENEFITS

- Consistency: Taking medication at the same time every day ensures stable blood sugar tiers.

- Effectiveness: Maximizes the effectiveness of the drugs.

TIPS

- Set Reminders: Use a pill organizer or set reminders on your telephone to make sure you don't forget about.
- Follow Prescriptions: Take medicinal drugs precisely as prescribed with the aid of your healthcare company.

4. Eat a Healthy Breakfast

Benefits

Blood Sugar Control: A balanced breakfast helps stabilize blood sugar ranges after a night time of fasting.

- Energy Boost: Provides the energy needed to begin the day and supports normal fitness.

IMPORTANCE OF BREAKFAST

The Importance of Breakfast for Diabetes Management

Eating a nutritious breakfast is a key thing of diabetes control. It helps modify blood sugar levels, provides important nutrients, and sets the level for healthful ingesting at some point of the day.

1. Blood Sugar Control

Prevents Blood Sugar Spikes

- Benefit: After a night of fasting, breakfast facilitates prevent a great rise in blood sugar tiers which can arise if you skip the morning meal.
- Outcome: Stabilizes blood sugar stages and presents a steady source of strength.

REDUCES INSULIN RESISTANCE

- Benefit: A balanced breakfast can enhance insulin sensitivity, making it less complicated for the body to apply insulin successfully.
- Outcome: Better blood sugar manipulate at some stage in the day.

2. Energy Boost

Provides Essential Nutrients

- Benefit: Breakfast affords vital vitamins like vitamins, minerals, protein, and

fiber which are essential for energy and
overall health.

- Outcome: Increases alertness and
cognitive function, helping you begin
your day with higher attention and
productivity.

Supports Physical Activity

- Benefit: Eating breakfast offers you the
power wished for bodily activities and
daily tasks.

- Outcome: Enhances performance in
morning exercise routines and other
sports.

3. Weight Management

Reduces Overeating

- Benefit: A wholesome breakfast can
help manage urge for food and decrease
the likelihood of overeating later inside
the day.

- Outcome: Supports weight control, which is vital for handling Type 2 diabetes.

Boosts Metabolism

- Benefit: Eating breakfast kick starts your metabolism, supporting your body burn energy extra successfully.

- Outcome: Promotes a healthy weight and improves average metabolic health.

4. Promotes Healthy Eating Habits

Establishes Routine

- Benefit: A ordinary breakfast routine encourages steady meal times and wholesome consuming behavior.

- Outcome: Helps keep solid blood sugar levels and supports normal dietary management.

Encourages Balanced Nutrition

- Benefit: A well planned breakfast consists of a mixture of carbohydrates, protein, and healthful fat, contributing to a balanced weight-reduction plan.

- Outcome: Ensures you start your day with the vitamins wished for most beneficial health.

5. Mental Health Benefits

Improves Mood

- Benefit: Consuming a nutritious breakfast can improve temper and reduce strain tiers.

- Outcome: Enhances mental well being, which is important for basic diabetes management.

Enhances Cognitive Function

- Benefit: Breakfast improves attention, reminiscence, and cognitive overall performance.

- Outcome: Helps you stay centered and efficient during the morning.

6. Supports Medication Effectiveness

Improves Medication Absorption

- Benefit: Some diabetes medicines are extra effective whilst occupied with meals.

- Outcome: Enhances the effectiveness of your medicine regimen and improves blood sugar manage.

Prevents Gastrointestinal Issues

- Benefit: Eating breakfast can save you nausea and different gastrointestinal problems that some diabetes medications may additionally purpose when taken on an empty stomach.

CHAPTER THREE: BALANCED DIET AND NUTRITION

UNDERSTANDING CARBOHYDRATES, PROTEINS, AND FATS

HOW DIFFERENT FOODS AFFECT BLOOD SUGAR LEVELS

Understanding how special meals affect blood sugar tiers is essential for effective diabetes management. Foods can effect blood sugar in various methods, relying on their composition and the price at which they may be digested and absorbed.

1. Carbohydrates

Simple Carbohydrates

- Sources: Sugary food and drinks, white bread, pastries, candy, and soda.

- Impact: Simple carbohydrates are fast digested and absorbed, inflicting speedy spikes in blood sugar degrees.

- Management Tip: Limit consumption of simple carbs and pick healthier alternatives to avoid unexpected blood sugar spikes.

Complex Carbohydrates

- Sources: Whole grains (brown rice, whole wheat bread, oats), legumes (beans, lentils), and starchy greens (sweet potatoes, corn).

- Impact: Complex carbohydrates are digested more slowly, leading to a gradual rise in blood sugar tiers.

- Management Tip: Include complicated carbs on your weight-reduction plan to maintain stable blood sugar ranges.

FIBERRICH CARBOHYDRATES

- Sources: Fruits, greens, entire grains, and legumes.

- Impact: Fiber slows down the digestion and absorption of carbohydrates, assisting to prevent fast blood sugar spikes.

- Management Tip: Aim to encompass high fiber foods in every meal to guide blood sugar control.

2. Proteins

Lean Proteins

- Sources: Poultry, fish, eggs, tofu, and low fat dairy merchandise.

- Impact: Proteins have a minimum direct effect on blood sugar degrees and can help stabilize blood sugar whilst eaten with carbohydrates.

- Management Tip: Incorporate lean proteins into food to decorate satiety and aid blood sugar manage.

High Fat Proteins

● Sources: Red meat, full fat dairy merchandise, and processed meats.

● Impact: High fat proteins can gradual digestion and doubtlessly lead to behind schedule blood sugar spikes.

● Management Tip: Choose lean protein resources and restrict intake of high fat proteins to promote higher blood sugar manipulate.

3. Fats

Healthy Fats

● Sources: Avocados, nuts, seeds, olive oil, and fatty fish (salmon, mackerel).

● Impact: Healthy fat have little direct impact on blood sugar stages and may help sluggish the absorption of carbohydrates.

● Management Tip: Include healthful fats on your food regimen to assist basic health and maintain strong blood sugar degrees.

UNHEALTHY FATS

- Sources: Fried ingredients, trans fat, and ingredients excessive in saturated fats (butter, lard).

- Impact: Unhealthy fats can contribute to insulin resistance and negatively impact blood sugar manipulate.

- Management Tip: Limit consumption of unhealthy fats and recognition on healthier fats assets.

4. GLYCEMIC Index (GI) and GLYCEMIC Load (GL)

GLYCEMIC INDEX (GI)

Definition: A degree of ways fast a carbohydrate containing food raises blood sugar degrees.

- Low GI Foods: Whole grains, legumes, most end result, and non starchy vegetables.

- High GI Foods: White bread, sugary cereals, and potatoes.

- Strategies for ingesting out and coping with blood sugar

- Strategies for Eating Out and Managing Blood Sugar

Eating out may be hard for individuals with diabetes, but with careful making plans and knowledgeable alternatives, it's viable to experience eating place food whilst preserving properly blood sugar manage.

1. Plan Ahead

Research Restaurants and Menus

- Benefit: Knowing the menu earlier lets in you to pick a eating place with diabetes friendly alternatives.

- Tips: Check the eating place's internet site or on-line critiques for menu alternatives. Look for dishes that consist of lean proteins, complete grains, and greens.

Eat a Small Snack

- Benefit: Eating a small, healthful snack earlier than going out can help manipulate starvation and prevent overeating.

- Tips: Choose a snack with protein and fiber, including a small handful of nuts or a chunk of fruit with cheese.

2. Make Smart Menu Choices

Opt for Grilled, Baked, or Steamed Foods

- Benefit: These cooking techniques generally contain less fat and fewer calories than fried or sauteed meals.

- Tips: Look for menu gadgets categorized as grilled, baked, or steamed and keep away from dishes defined as crispy, fried, or sauteed.

CHOOSE WHOLE GRAINS

- Benefit: Whole grains have a decrease glycemic index (GI) and provide more fiber than subtle grains.

- Tips: Ask if complete grain alternatives like brown rice, entire wheat bread, or quinoa are to be had.

Load Up on Vegetables

- Benefit: Vegetables are low in calories and carbohydrates however high in fiber and vitamins.

- Tips: Order a side salad or extra greens along with your meal. Opt for non starchy vegetables like broccoli, spinach, or bell peppers.

BE CAUTIOUS WITH SAUCES AND DRESSINGS

- Benefit: Many sauces and dressings are high in sugar and unhealthy fat.

- Tips: Request sauces and dressings on the aspect so you can manage the amount. Choose oil and vinegar or ask for light dressings.

3. Control Portions

Share or Save Half

- Benefit: Restaurant portions are frequently large than what you need, leading to overeating.

- Tips: Share a meal with a friend or ask for a togo field when your food arrives and shop 1/2 for another meal.

ORDER APPETIZERS OR SIDE DISHES

- Benefit: Appetizers and side dishes are normally smaller in component size.

- Tips: Choose an appetizer or two side dishes in place of a complete entree.

4. Mind Your Beverages

Choose Water or Unsweetened Beverages

- Benefit: Sugary beverages can cause fast spikes in blood sugar levels.

- Tips: Drink water, unsweetened tea, or espresso. If you pick a flavored drink, ask for water with a touch of lemon or lime.

Limit Alcohol Intake

- Benefit: Alcohol can affect blood sugar degrees and have interaction with diabetes medications.

- Tips: If you pick out to drink, limit yourself to 1 drink in keeping with day for girls and for men. Opt for dry wines or spirits with out a introduced sugar, and always drink with meals.

5. Be Prepared to Manage Blood Sugar

Monitor Blood Sugar Levels

- Benefit: Knowing your blood sugar degrees before and after food enables you recognize how exceptional ingredients have an effect on you.

- Tips: Carry your blood glucose meter with you and test your degrees as endorsed via your healthcare issuer.

Carry Supplies

- Benefit: Having your diabetes supplies on hand ensures you may manage any unexpected changes in blood sugar degrees.

- Tips: Bring your blood glucose meter, check strips, insulin, or different medicines, and a few fast acting glucose (like glucose tablets or a small juice field) in case of low blood sugar.

6. Communicate Your Needs

Inform the Server

- Benefit: Letting the server realize you have nutritional regulations can help ensure your meal meets your needs.

- Tips: Politely give an explanation for any dietary restrictions and ask for changes to menu items if important. Don't hesitate to invite questions about how the food is ready.

CUSTOMIZE YOUR ORDER

- Benefit: Customizing your meal allows you to control what you consume and the way it affects your blood sugar.

- Tips: Request substitutions, consisting of a facet salad rather than fries, or ask for food to be organized with much less oil or butter.

HOW TO STAY ADEQUATELY HYDRATED

Staying hydrated is vital for ordinary health and mainly crucial for people managing diabetes, as right hydration enables adjust blood sugar tiers.

1. Understand Your Hydration Needs

Daily Water Intake

General Guideline: Aim for about eight glasses (sixty four oz.) of water in line with day, but man or woman needs may range based on elements inclusive of age, weight, hobby degree, and weather.

- Specific Needs: People with diabetes may also need to display their hydration greater closely, mainly if experiencing high blood sugar levels, that may increase the risk of dehydration.

LISTEN TO YOUR BODY

- Thirst: Thirst is a clear signal that your frame needs water. Don't ignore it.

- Other Signs: Dark yellow urine, dry mouth, fatigue, dizziness, and confusion can also indicate dehydration.

2. Drink Water Throughout the Day

REGULAR INTERVALS

- Set Reminders: Use a telephone app or a timer to remind you to drink water frequently.

- Routine: Incorporate drinking water into your daily routine, consisting of having a pitcher with every meal and snack.

CARRY A WATER BOTTLE

- Accessibility: Keep a reusable water bottle with you at all times to make it smooth to drink water at some stage in the day.

- Measurement: Choose a bottle with measurements at the side to track your intake.

3. Enhance Your Water

FLAVOR ENHANCERS

Natural Additives: Add slices of lemon, lime, cucumber, or clean mint for your water for a refreshing taste with out brought sugars.

Infused Water: Prepare infused water by using including end result and herbs to a glass and letting it take a seat within the refrigerator for some hours.

COLD OR WARM WATER

- Preference: Drink water at a temperature you find maximum enjoyable, whether it's cold, room temperature, or heat, to inspire greater frequent consumption.

4. Incorporate Hydrating Foods

High Water Content Foods

- Fruits: Watermelon, strawberries, cantaloupe, oranges, and grapefruit.

- Vegetables: Cucumbers, lettuce, celery, zucchini, and bell peppers.

- Benefit: These ingredients no longer most effective contribute for your ordinary fluid consumption but additionally provide important vitamins and minerals.

Broths and Soups

- Hydration and Nutrition: Soups and broths are awesome approaches to boom fluid intake even as additionally getting vitamins.

- Low Sodium Options: Choose low sodium types to keep away from excess salt consumption.

5. Limit Dehydrating Beverages

Caffeinated Drinks

- Moderation: While slight caffeine intake may be a part of a healthful diet, excessive intake can cause dehydration. Balance caffeinated liquids like coffee and tea with water intake.

- Decaf Options: Consider decaffeinated versions of your preferred beverages to reduce caffeine intake.

Sugary and Alcoholic Beverages

- Avoidance: Sugary beverages and alcohol can dehydrate your frame and affect blood sugar tiers. Limit consumption and compensate with extra water.

6. Monitor Hydration in Different Conditions

Exercise and Physical Activity

- Pre Hydrate: Drink water earlier than beginning any physical pastime.

- During Exercise: Sip water at regular intervals for the duration of your workout.

- Post Exercise: Replenish fluids misplaced via sweat by using consuming water after workout.

Hot Weather

Increased Needs: In hot or humid climate, your frame loses greater water thru sweat. Increase your water consumption to stay hydrated.

Illness

Fever, Vomiting, and Diarrhea: These situations can result in sizeable fluid loss. Drink greater fluids and take into account oral re hydration solutions if necessary.

CHAPTER FOUR: EXERCISE AND PHYSICAL ACTIVITY

BENEFITS OF REGULAR EXERCISE

IMPACT OF PHYSICAL ACTIVITY ON BLOOD SUGAR LEVELS

Physical interest plays a giant function in dealing with diabetes and retaining general fitness. It immediately impacts blood sugar stages, insulin sensitivity, and typical glucose metabolism.

1. Immediate Effects on Blood Sugar Levels

Glucose Utilization

- Increased Muscle Activity: During exercise, muscle groups use greater glucose for energy, main to a lower in blood sugar tiers.

- Immediate Reduction: Moderate to extreme bodily activity can decrease

blood sugar stages right now and for
several hours post exercise.

Insulin Sensitivity

- Enhanced Sensitivity: Exercise will increase insulin sensitivity, meaning your frame's cells are greater effective at the usage of available insulin to take in glucose at some stage in and after pastime.

- Benefit: This effect can last up to 48 hours, enhancing average blood sugar control.

Hormonal Changes

- Hormone Release: Physical interest triggers the discharge of hormones like adrenaline and glucagon, which can increase blood sugar degrees temporarily, specially in the course of high intensity exercise.

- Balance: The typical effect has a tendency to decrease blood sugar levels as glucose is used by muscle groups.

2. Long Term Benefits

Improved Glycemic Control

- Regular Activity: Consistent bodily hobby allows preserve decrease blood sugar degrees through the years.

- A1C Reduction: Regular workout can result in reductions in HbA1c stages, a key marker of long term blood sugar control.

Weight Management

- Calorie Burning: Exercise enables burn calories, contributing to weight reduction or upkeep.

- Reduced Insulin Resistance: Weight loss, specifically the discount of visceral fats, can improve insulin sensitivity and reduce insulin resistance.

Cardiovascular Health

- Heart Health: Physical interest strengthens the heart and improves circulation, that's crucial for human beings with diabetes who are at better risk for cardiovascular sickness.

- Blood Pressure: Regular workout can assist lower blood strain and improve typical cardiovascular health.

3. Types of Exercise and Their Effects

Aerobic Exercise

Examples: Walking, strolling, cycling, swimming.

- Impact: Typically lowers blood sugar levels greater quickly during and after the pastime. Helps enhance cardiovascular health and average glucose metabolism.

Resistance Training

- Examples: Weight lifting, resistance band exercises, body weight physical games.

- Impact: Builds muscle mass, which increases the body's capacity to store glucose and improves insulin sensitivity. Leads to more solid blood sugar stages over time.

- Flexibility and Balance Exercises

- Examples: Yoga, tai chi.

- Impact: While no longer without delay affecting blood sugar levels as extensively as aerobic or resistance sporting events, these activities lessen strain and enhance typical well being, indirectly supporting blood sugar management.

High Intensity Interval Training (HIIT)

 Examples: Short bursts of intense exercising accompanied by relaxation or low intensity exercise.

● Impact: Can hastily decrease blood sugar tiers and improve insulin sensitivity. May reason transient spikes in blood sugar because of hormonal responses, however normal blessings outweigh transient increases.

4. Exercise Considerations for Managing Blood Sugar

Monitoring Blood Sugar Levels

● Before Exercise: Check blood sugar ranges to make sure they're no longer too low (below one hundred mg/dL) or too excessive (above 250 mg/dL) before starting bodily interest.

● During Exercise: Be aware about signs of hypoglycemia (low blood sugar) together with shakiness, dizziness, or confusion, and feature fast acting carbohydrates (like glucose tablets) reachable.

- After Exercise: Monitor blood sugar levels to apprehend how different types and intervals of exercise affect your levels.

Adjusting Food and Medication

- Carbohydrate Intake: Consume a small carbohydrate rich snack if blood sugar stages are low before beginning exercising.

- Medication Adjustments: Consult together with your healthcare issuer approximately adjusting insulin or other diabetes medicinal drugs to prevent hypoglycemia at some stage in or after exercising.

Hydration

- Stay Hydrated: Drink lots of water before, for the duration of, and after exercising to prevent dehydration, that can have an effect on blood sugar degrees.

Consistent Routine

- Regular Schedule: Establish a regular exercising habitual to assist keep strong blood sugar ranges and enhance overall fitness.

Types of Exercise

Certainly! There are several types of sporting events, each presenting unique blessings for bodily fitness, common health, and dealing with conditions like diabetes.

1. Aerobic Exercises (Cardiovascular Exercise)

Examples:

- Walking
- Jogging/Running
- Cycling
- Swimming
- Dancing

Aerobics lessons

Benefits:

- Improves cardiovascular health by using strengthening the heart and lungs.
- Helps burn calories and aids in weight management.
- Increases persistence and stamina.
- Lowers blood strain and decreases the risk of heart disorder.
- Can enhance mood and decrease pressure.

2. Resistance Training (Strength Training)

Examples:

- Weight lifting
- Body weight physical activities (push ups, squats, lunges)
- Resistance band exercises
- Using weight machines

Benefits:

- Builds muscle power and mass.

- Improves bone density and reduces the chance of osteoporosis.
- Boosts metabolism, helping with weight management.
- Enhances functional power for every day sports.
- Can improve insulin sensitivity and blood sugar manipulate.

3. Flexibility and Stretching Exercises

Examples:

- Yoga
- Pilates
- Stretching workouts

Benefits:

- Increases flexibility and variety of movement in joints.
- Improves posture and balance.
- Reduces the hazard of accidents.
- Can relieve muscle tension and improve rest.

- Enhances usual mobility and physical function.

4. High Intensity Interval Training (HIIT)

Examples:

- Sprint duration's
- Circuit schooling
- Tabatha exercises

Benefits:

- Burns calories correctly and promotes weight reduction.
- Improves cardiovascular health and endurance.
- Increases metabolic price even after exercise (post exercise oxygen intake).
- Enhances insulin sensitivity and glucose metabolism.
- Time efficient workout routines due to high depth.

5. Balance and Stability Exercises

Examples:

- Tai Chi

- Balance physical activities (status on one leg, stroll)
- Stability ball physical activities

HOW TO CONTAIN EXERCISE INTO DAY BY DAY EXISTENCE

Incorporating workout into daily life does not must be complex.

1. Set Realistic Goals

Start Small:

- Begin with practicable dreams, together with 10 minutes of exercising per day.
- Gradually increase the period and depth as you construct stamina and self assurance.

Specific Objectives:

Define clear and specific workout goals, along with strolling for 30 minutes 5 days every week or completing a power education consultation two times every week.

2. Choose Activities You Enjoy

Find What You Like:

- Select sports which you find enjoyable and tasty, whether it is dancing, swimming, biking, or gambling a recreation.

- Variety keeps things thrilling and forestalls boredom.

Make it Social:

Exercise with buddies, circle of relatives participants, or be part of organization fitness classes to make exercises extra enjoyable and motivating.

3. Make It a Priority

Schedule Your Workouts:

- Treat exercise like an crucial appointment by using scheduling it into your daily calendar.

- Choose a time of day while you're most likely to paste in your ordinary (e.G., morning, lunch smash, nighttime).

Consistency is Key:

Aim for consistency as opposed to depth. Regular, mild exercise is extra sustainable than sporadic, excessive workouts.

4. Incorporate Activity into Daily Tasks

Active Commuting:

- Walk, bike, or use public transportation instead of riding whenever viable.
- If driving is necessary, park farther far from your vacation spot to get extra steps.

Break Time Movement:

Take brief hobby breaks at some stage in the day. Stand up, stretch, stroll around, or do a short workout recurring at your table.

5. Make Use of Technology

Fitness Apps:

- Use cellphone apps to song your workout routines, set reminders, and get entry to workout routines.

- Many apps provide guided exercises, progress tracking, and motivation capabilities.

Wearable Devices:

- Consider the use of fitness trackers or smartwatches to reveal your interest stages, coronary heart charge, and sleep patterns.
- Set each day step dreams or interest targets to maintain you stimulated.

6. Involve Family and Friends

Family Activities:

- Include physical sports in own family time, such as hiking, cycling, gambling out of doors games, or going for walks together.
- Make workout a fun and bonding experience for each person.

Accountability Partners:

- Partner with a friend, member of the family, or colleague for normal exercises or challenges.
- Accountability and assist can hold you inspired and on the right track.

7. Be Flexible and Listen to Your Body

Adapt to Changes:

- Be flexible together with your workout routine to house adjustments in time table, climate, or non-public options.
- Have opportunity indoor and outside activities ready for specific conditions.

Listen to Your Body:

- Pay attention to how your body feels in the course of and after exercising.
- Rest and recover whilst wished, and don't push your self too difficult if you're now not feeling nicely.

STAYING ACTIVE WITH A BUSY SCHEDULE

Staying active with a hectic agenda may be tough, but it's really feasible with some strategic making plans and prioritization.

1. Prioritize Exercise

- Schedule Workouts: Treat workout as an essential appointment through scheduling it into your calendar. Choose a time that works excellent for you, whether or not it's early morning, for the duration of lunch ruin, or inside the evening.

- Make It Non Negotiable: Commit for your exercise periods as you would to another critical undertaking. Avoid canceling or rescheduling unless actually necessary.

2. Choose Efficient Workouts

- High Intensity Interval Training (HIIT): HIIT workouts are short however effective, combining bursts of excessive exercising with periods of relaxation. They may be completed in as little as 1530 mins and offer great cardiovascular and metabolic benefits.

- Circuit Training: Circuit exercises contain moving from one exercise to another with minimal relaxation in among. They target a couple of muscle corporations and offer a full body exercising in a quick quantity of time.

- Tabatha Workouts: Tabatha education consists of 20 seconds of severe workout accompanied by 10 seconds of relaxation, repeated for more than one rounds. It's a time efficient way to improve cardiovascular health and burn energy.

3. Incorporate Activity Into Daily Tasks

Active Commuting: If possible, stroll, motorbike, or use public transportation instead of driving to work or close by destinations.

- Take Breaks: Use quick breaks at some point of the day to stretch, do brief physical games, or take a brisk walk. This can help break up sedentary duration's and raise energy ranges.

- Use Stairs: Opt for stairs instead of elevators each time viable. Climbing stairs is a wonderful manner to sneak in a few extra physical interest.

4. Make Use of Technology

- Fitness Apps: Use health apps to get admission to brief workout routines, song your pastime ranges, set reminders, and live stimulated. Many apps offer guided exercises that may be executed at home or in constrained area.

- Wearable Devices: Consider using a health tracker or smartwatch to screen your each day steps, interest tiers, and typical progress. Set each day activity desires to keep your self accountable.

5. Incorporate Activity Into Daily Routines

- Active Lunch Breaks: Use your lunch damage to take a walk, do yoga stretches, or interact in other bodily activities. Invite coworkers to enroll in you for a walking assembly or lunchtime exercise.

- Family Activities: Plan energetic outings or own family sports on weekends or evenings, which includes hiking, cycling, gambling sports, or traveling a park. It's a top notch way to bond with loved ones at the same time as staying active.

- Home Workouts: Invest in some primary exercising gadget like dumbbells, resistance bands, or a yoga mat. You can

do brief workouts at home whilst time is
limited.

6. Stay Motivated and Consistent

- Set Goals: Establish realistic health
goals that align with your time table and
way of life. Track your progress and
celebrate milestones along the manner.

- Find Accountability: Partner with a
workout pal, be part of a fitness
magnificence, or lease a private
instructor for introduced accountability
and motivation.

- Be Flexible: Life may be unpredictable,
so be bendy with your workout recurring.
If you leave out a exercising or have a
hectic day, don't get discouraged.
Resume your recurring day after today
and stay consistent.

7. Focus on Efficiency and Enjoyment

- Choose Activities You Enjoy: Find bodily activities which you truly revel in, whether it's dancing, trekking, swimming, or working towards yoga. You're much more likely to stay with a exercise routine if it brings you satisfaction.

TIPS FOR BECOMING IN BODILY ACTIVITY DURING THE DAY.

1. Schedule It

- Prioritize Exercise: Treat bodily activity as a nonnegotiable a part of your every day agenda.

- Set Reminders: Use alarms or calendar notifications to remind your self to move at some point of the day.

- Plan Ahead: Schedule workouts or hobby breaks in advance to make sure they match into your day.

2. Break It Up

- Short Bursts: Fit in short bursts of activity at some stage in the day, including 10minute walks, stretching breaks, or mini workout routines.

- Micro Workouts: Break longer workout routines into shorter sessions if time is confined. For instance, do 3 10minute exercises as opposed to one 30minute consultation.

- Activity Snacks: Think of bodily hobby as "snacks" that you can sprinkle all through your day for power and rejuvenation.

3. Be Efficient

Choose High Intensity Workouts: Opt for activities that offer most benefits in minimum time, including HIIT workouts, circuit schooling, or Tabata duration's.

Multitask Mindfully: Combine bodily activity with other duties when feasible, inclusive of on foot conferences, status while on cellphone calls, or doing squats even as brushing your tooth.

4. Incorporate Movement Into Daily Tasks

Active Commuting: Walk, bike, or use public transportation for part of your go back and forth.

- Take the Stairs: Use stairs in preference to elevators whenever feasible.

- Active Breaks: Stand up, stretch, or do a brief workout recurring at some point of breaks at work or even as studying.

5. Make It Fun and Social

- Choose Enjoyable Activities: Find bodily activities which you enjoy, whether or not it's dancing, gambling a recreation, hiking, or training yoga.

- Involve Others: Exercise with buddies, circle of relatives participants, or coworkers for motivation and social interaction.

- Try New Things: Keep your exercises exciting through trying new sports or lessons to prevent boredom.

6. Use Technology and Apps

Fitness Trackers: Use a fitness tracker or cellphone app to screen your pastime degrees, set desires, and tune development.

- Exercise Apps: Explore workout apps that offer guided exercises, customization workouts, and motivation capabilities.

- Mindfulness Apps: Consider mindfulness apps that encompass motion or stretching sporting activities for relaxation and strain remedy.

7. Prioritize Self Care

- Make Time: Recognize the importance of self care and bodily interest in keeping normal health.

- Set Boundaries: Establish barriers to shield your exercise time and prioritize your health.

- Celebrate Achievements: Acknowledge and have a good time your efforts and achievements in becoming physical interest into your day.